P is for Poo

By

Ms. Butterfly

Illustrated by

Ms. Butterfly

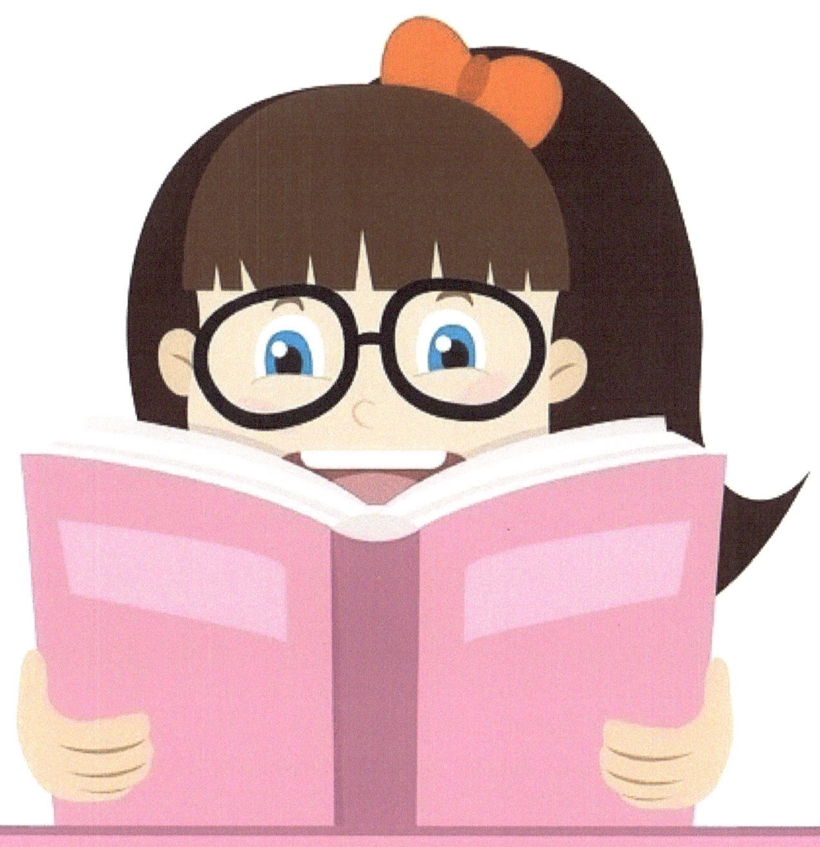

This book belongs to

Dedication

I would like to dedicate this book to all the children in the world that love books and love learning to read. Enjoy your studies and always try your best!

Love Ms. Butterfly

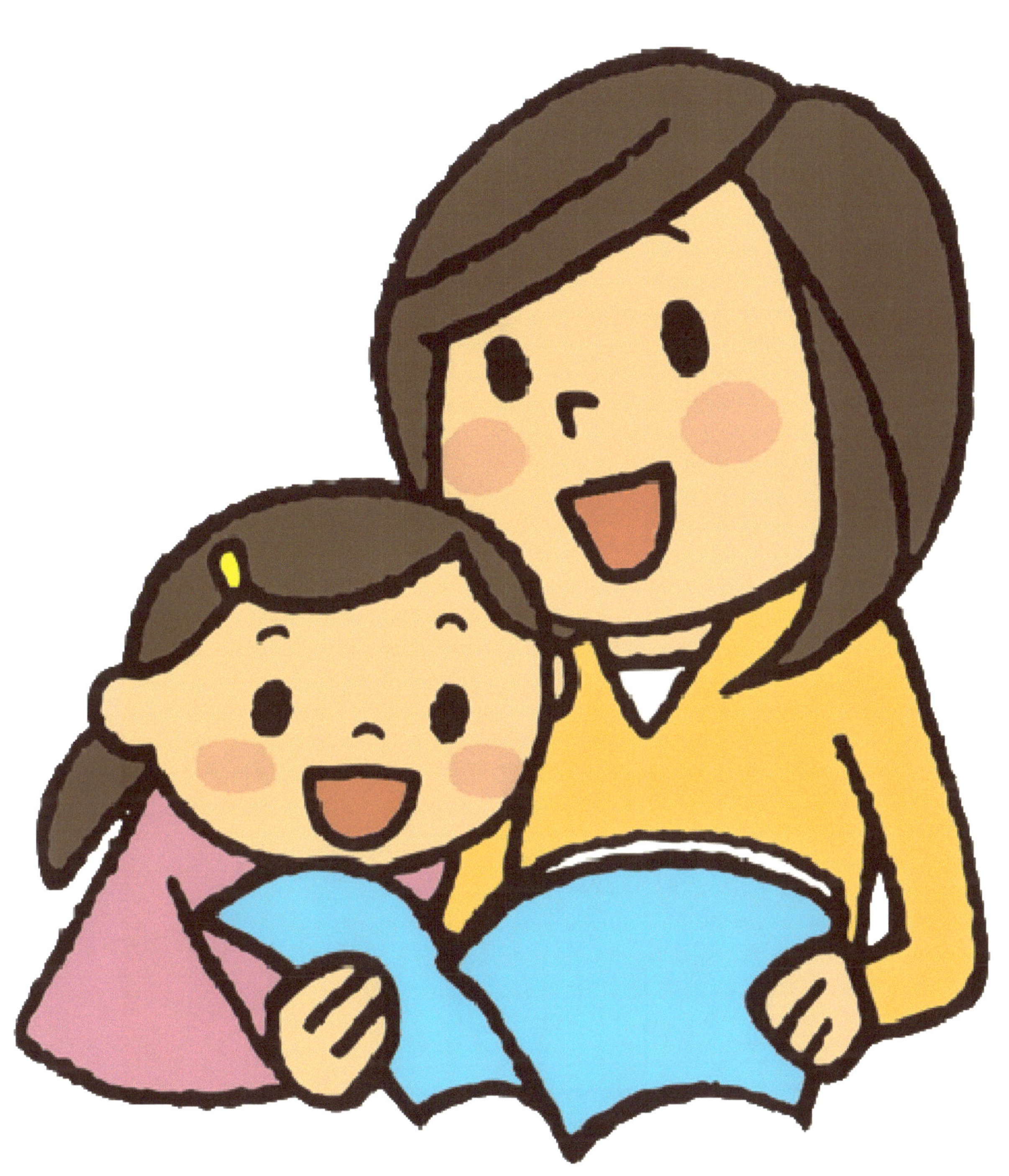

Pooping is good for you because food that you eat is digested and your body gets nutrients. The food that you don't need becomes poo.

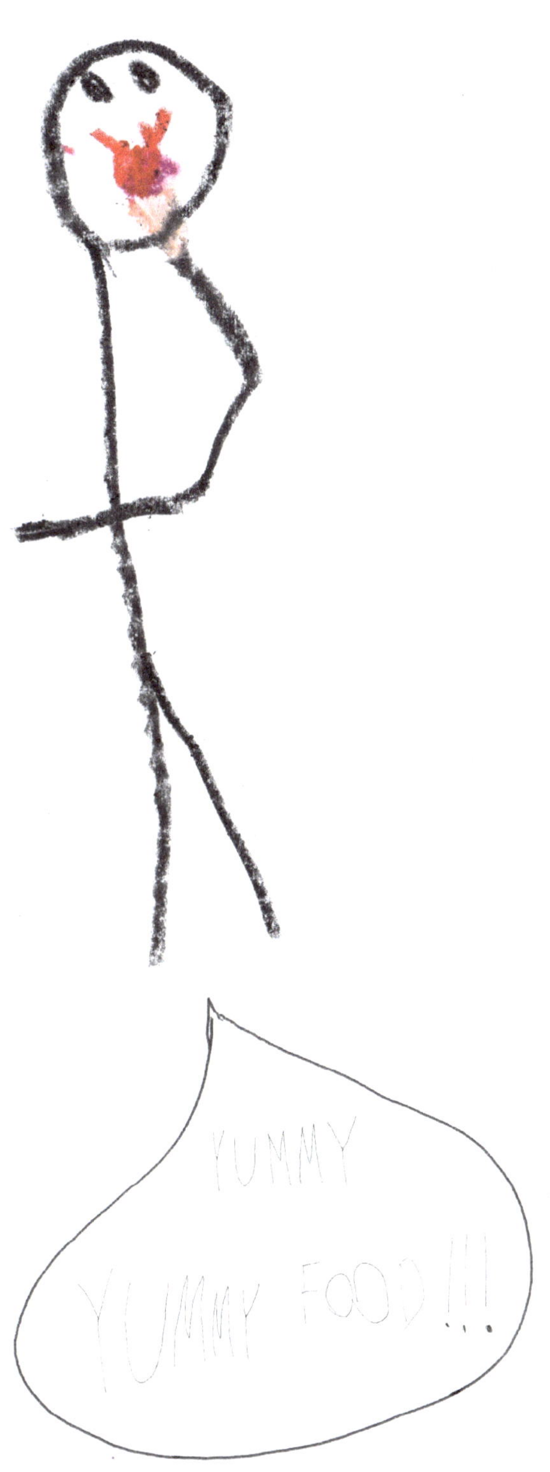
YUMMY
YUMMY FOOD!!!
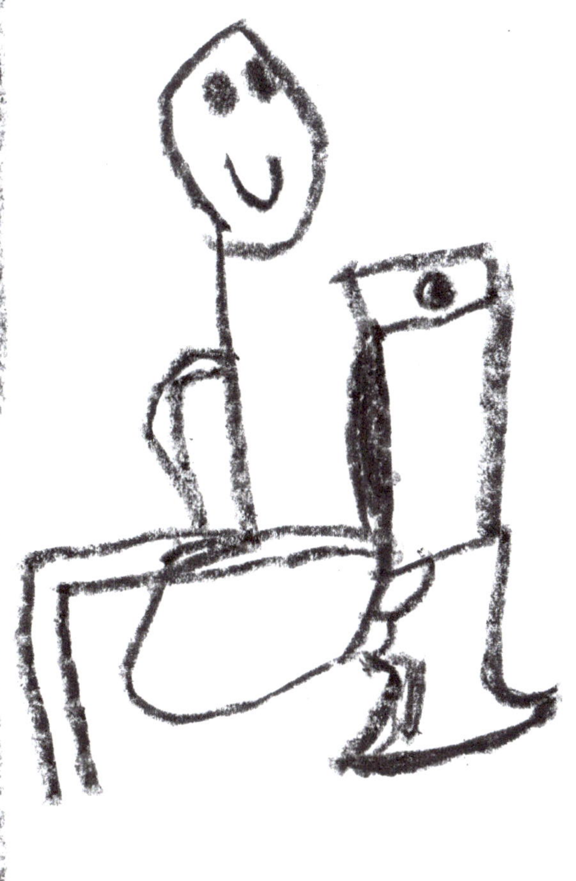

If you don't poo then you become constipated and you can get sick. Sometimes you can vomit and be in lots of pain.

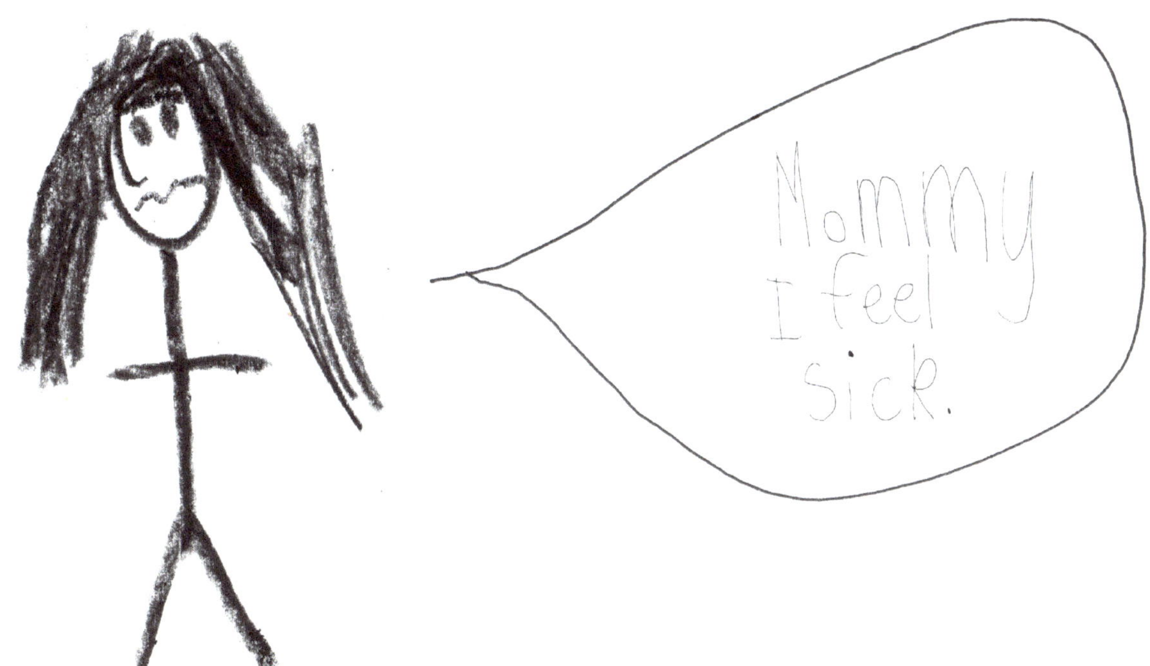

Mommy I feel sick.

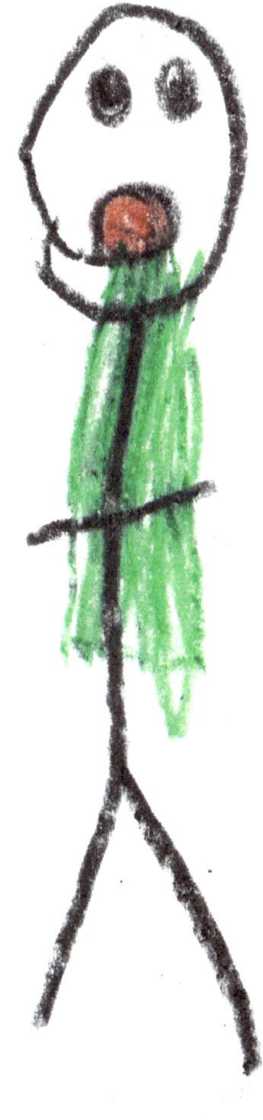

BBBLLLAAARRRGGGHHH !!!

My little sister was constipated so we gave her 'P' fruits so she could poo.

Maybe these fruits can help your baby too!

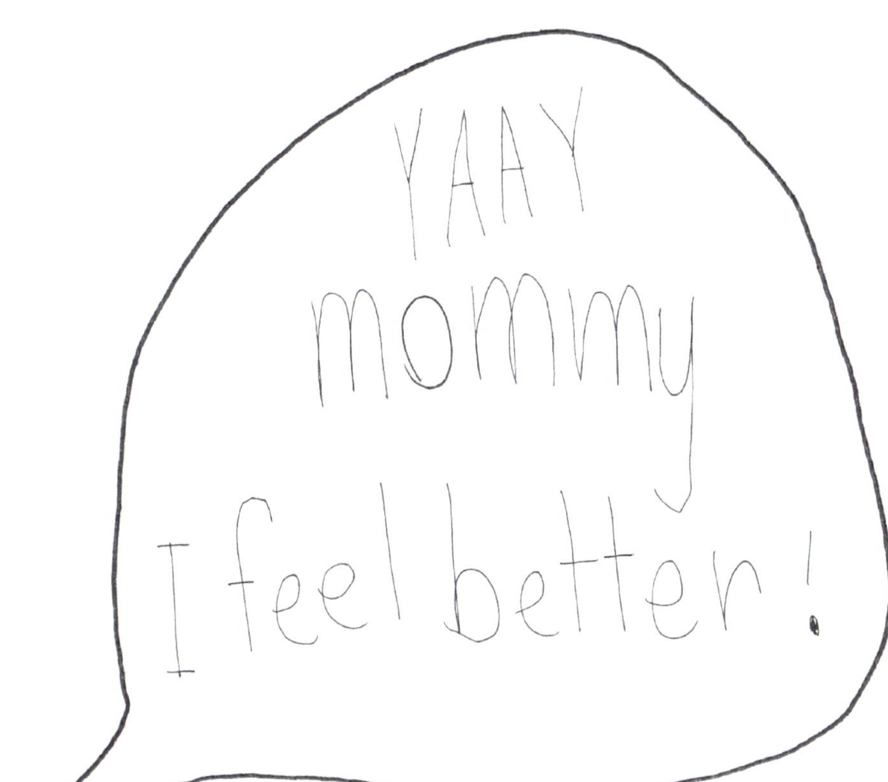
YAAY
mommy
I feel better!

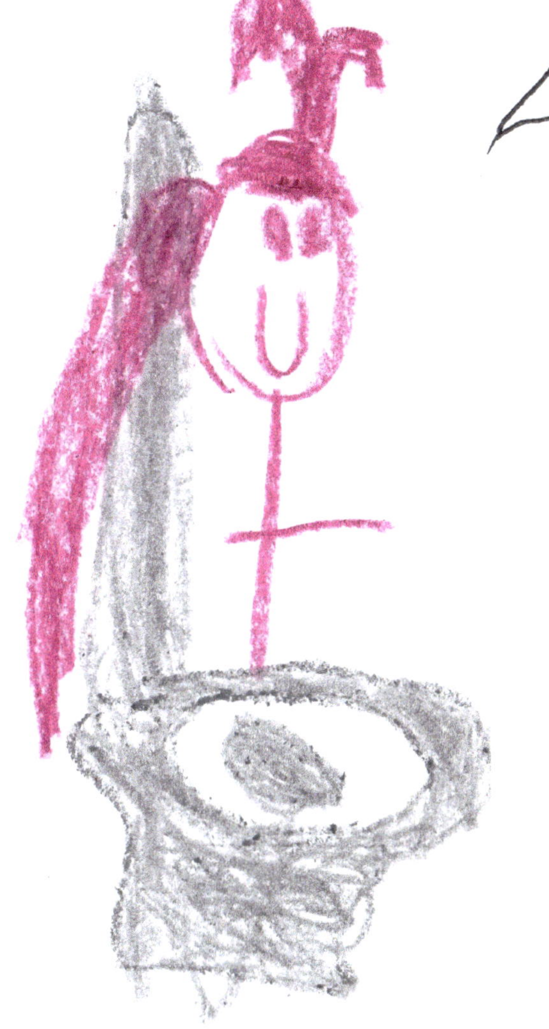

This is a pear.
You can definately
make cool smoothies
with this fruit.

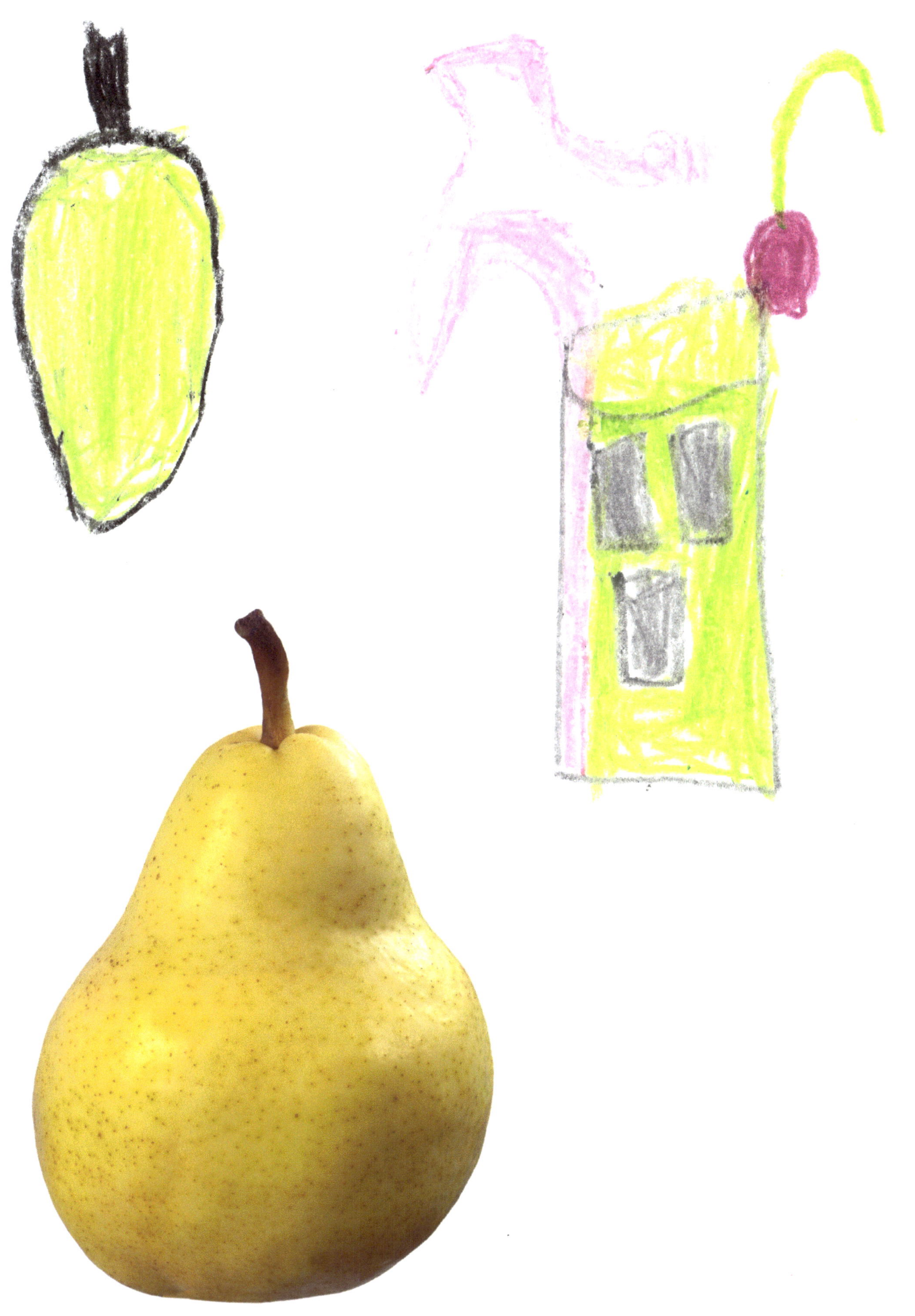

This is a peach.

It is great for eating

on its own and

peaches are delicious.

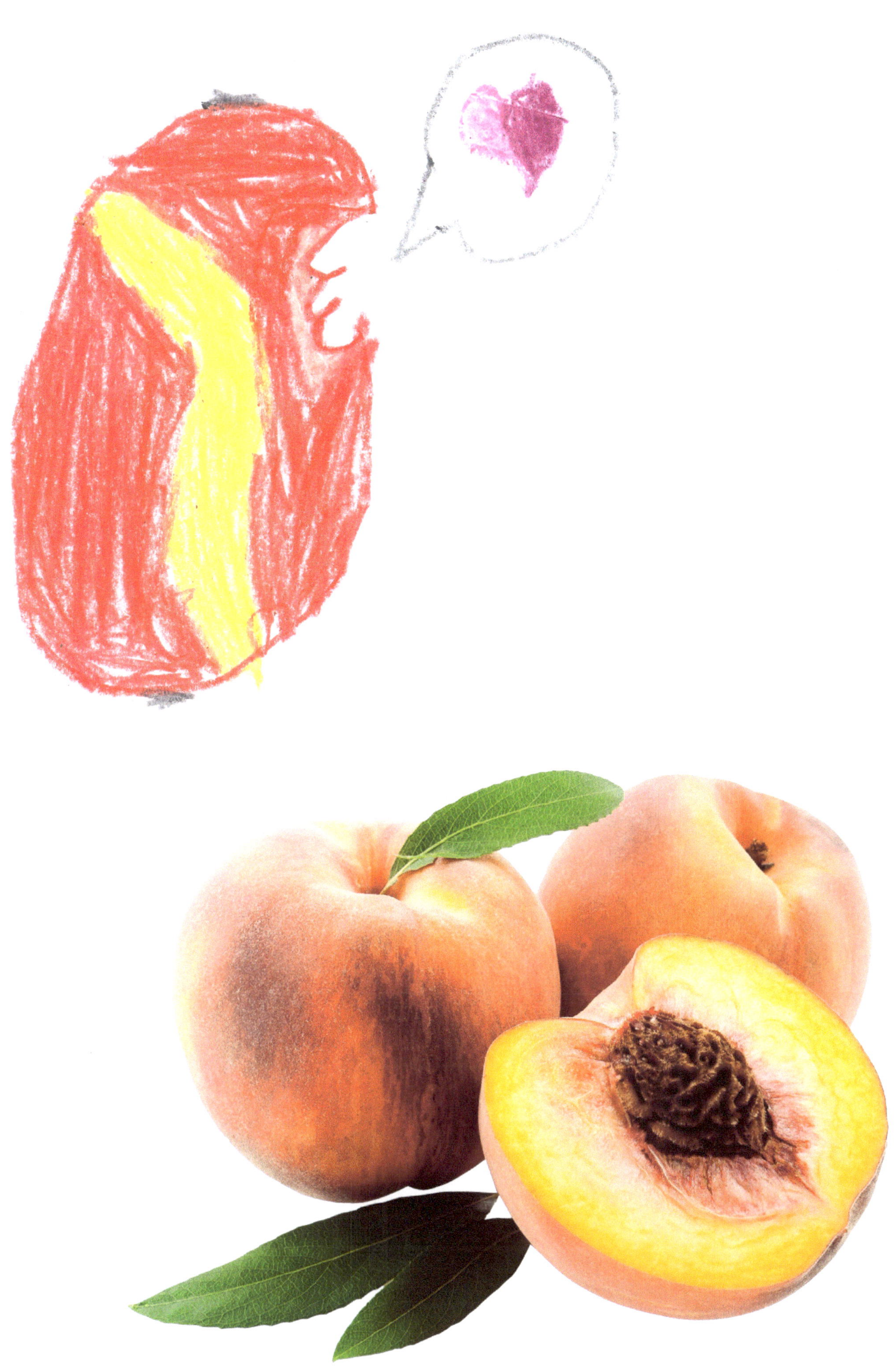

This is a papaya. It is a very soft orange-colored fruit that tastes like a melon. When I was little I loved eating it. YUM YUM YUM!!!

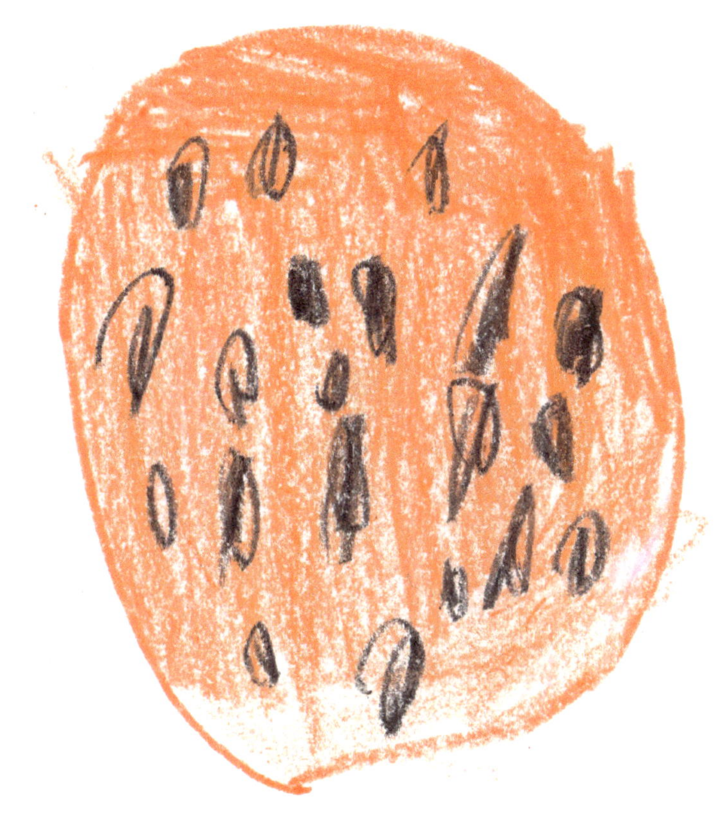

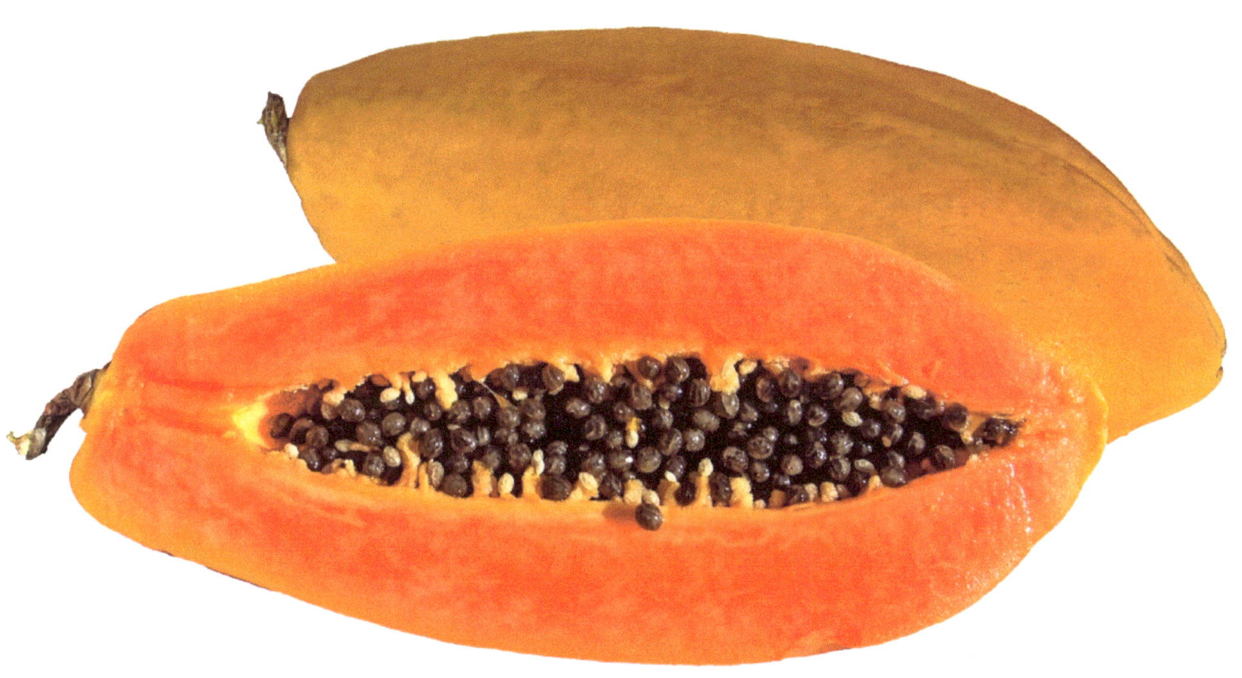

This is a prune.
We can make cupcakes
with it or drink

prune juice!

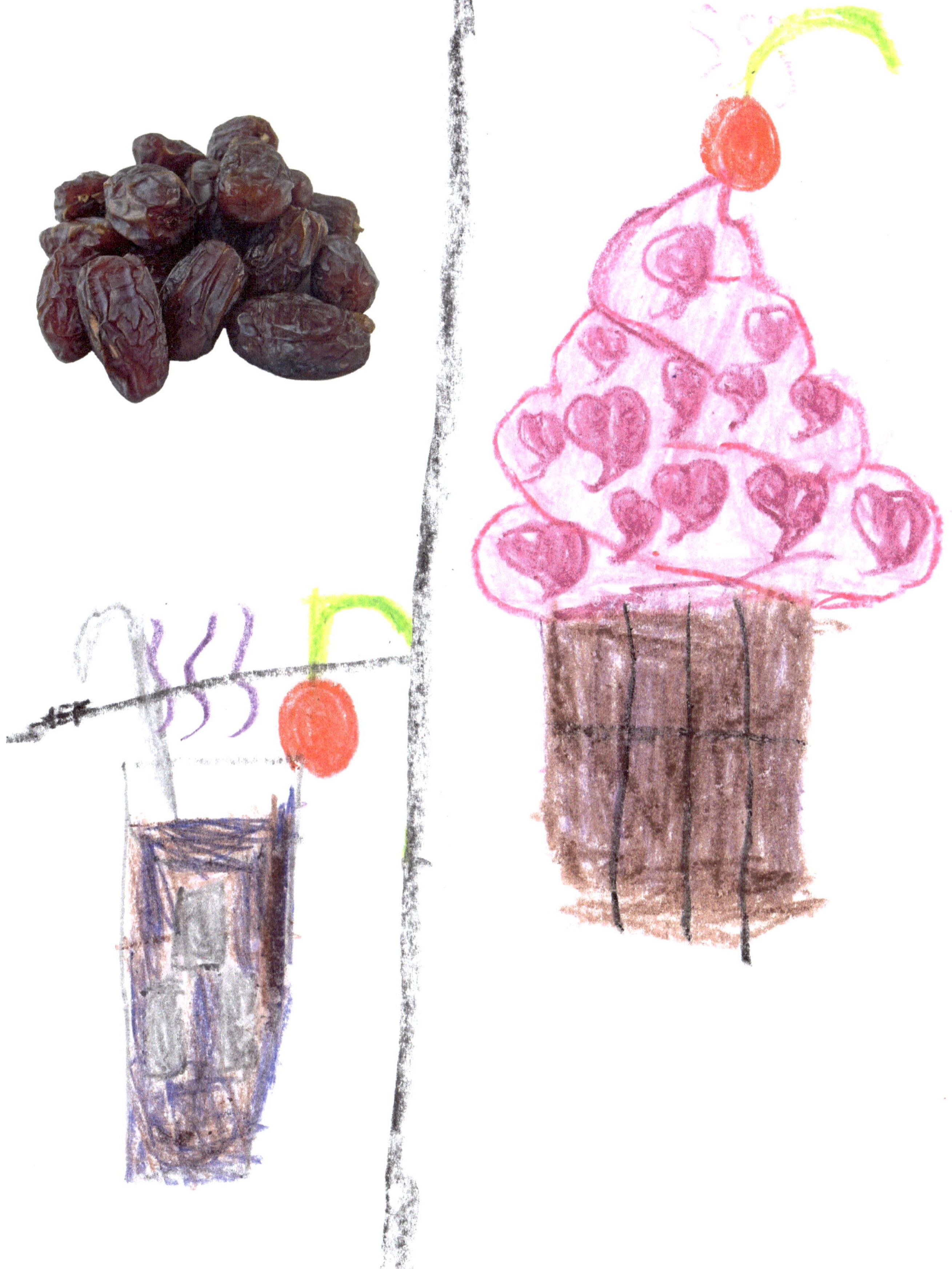

This is a pomegranate It is round and red.

You need to eat two cups of its seeds per day!

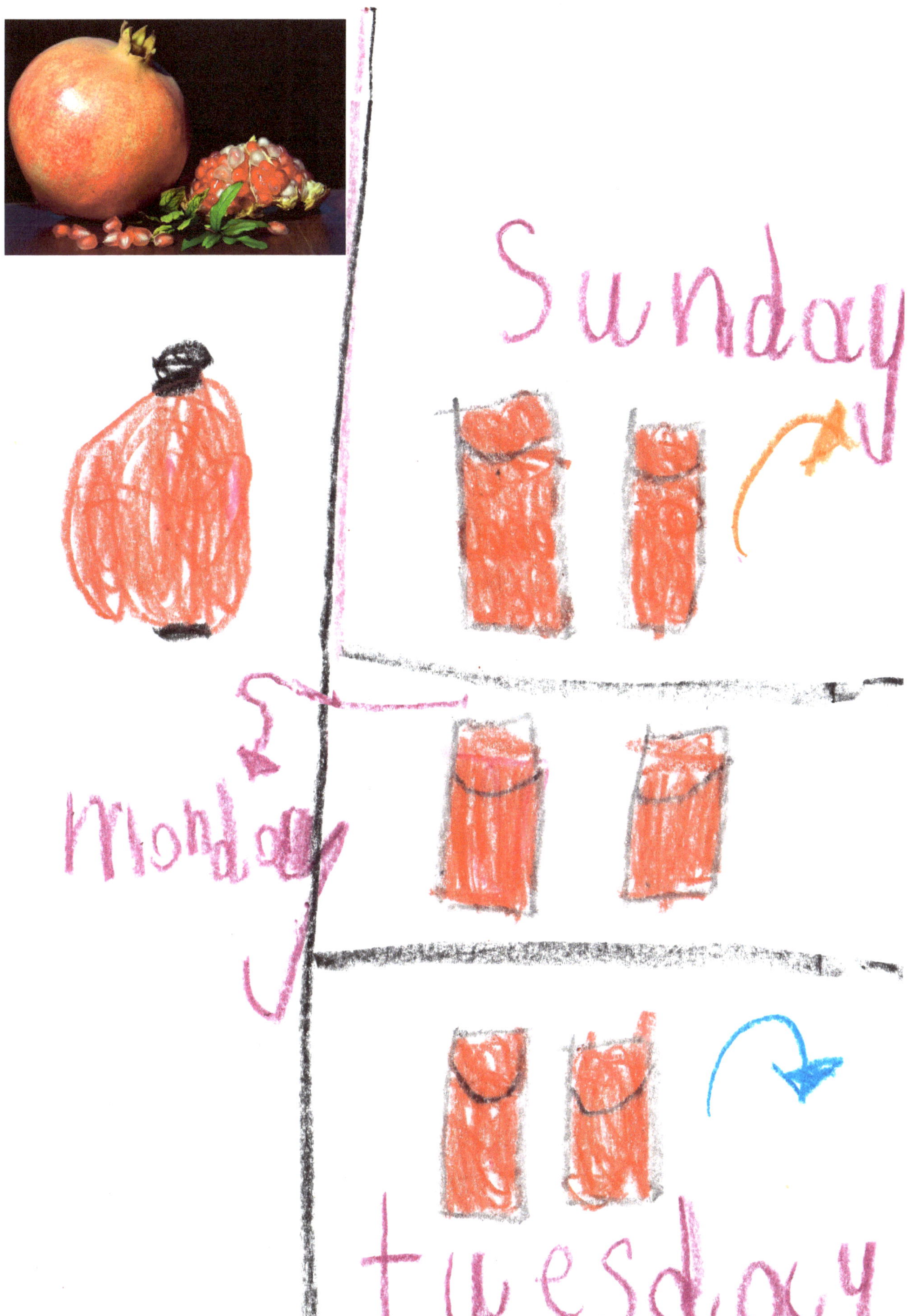

Sunday
Monday
tuesday

All of these fruit help with constipation and are very healthy for you.

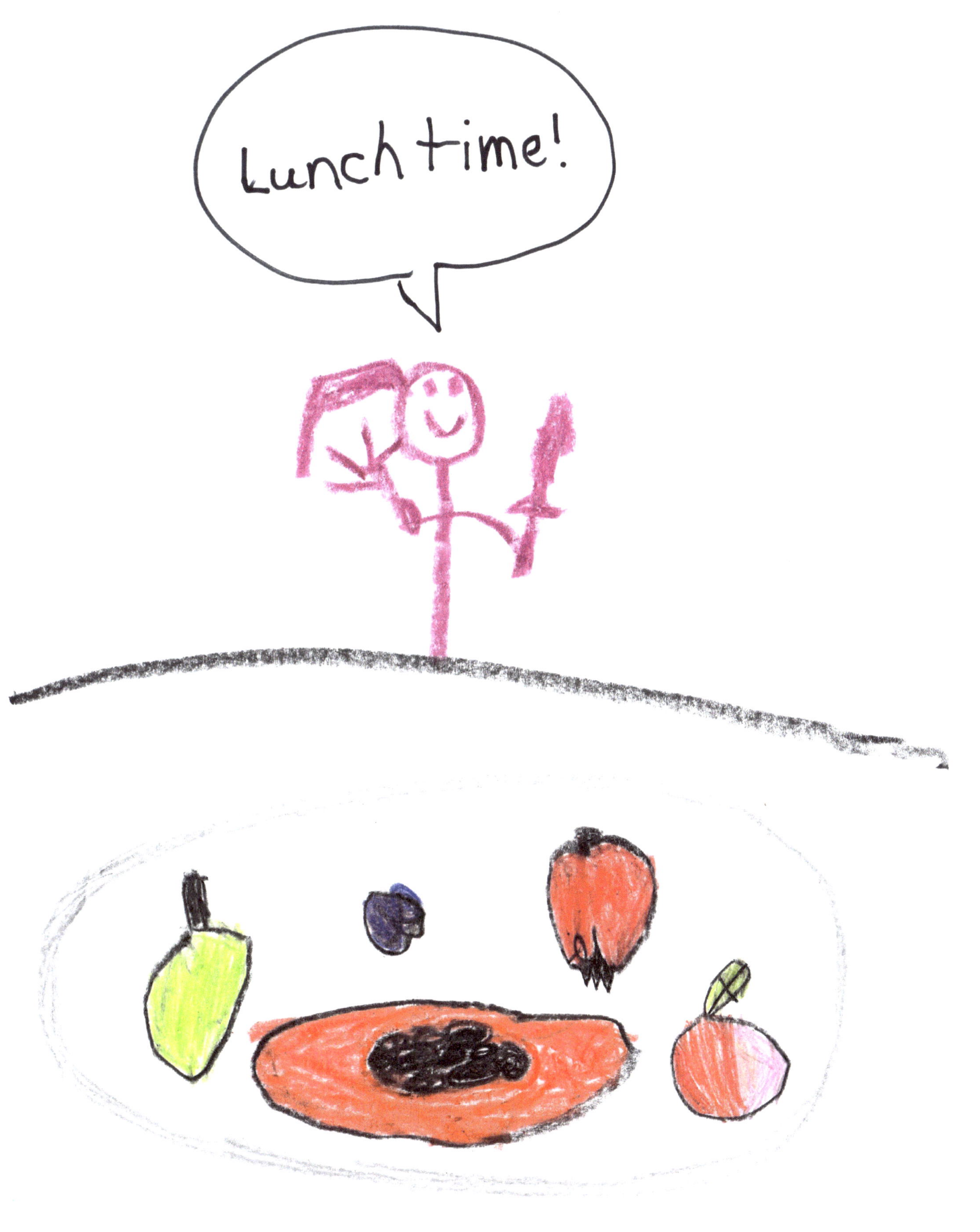
Lunch time!

THE END

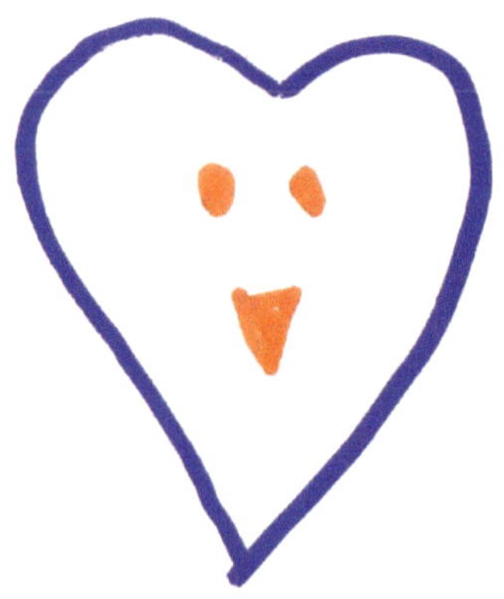

Thank you for reading.

I hope you enjoyed the story.

On the following pages you will find some fruit coloring activities.

Let's all practise together.

Love Ms. Butterfly

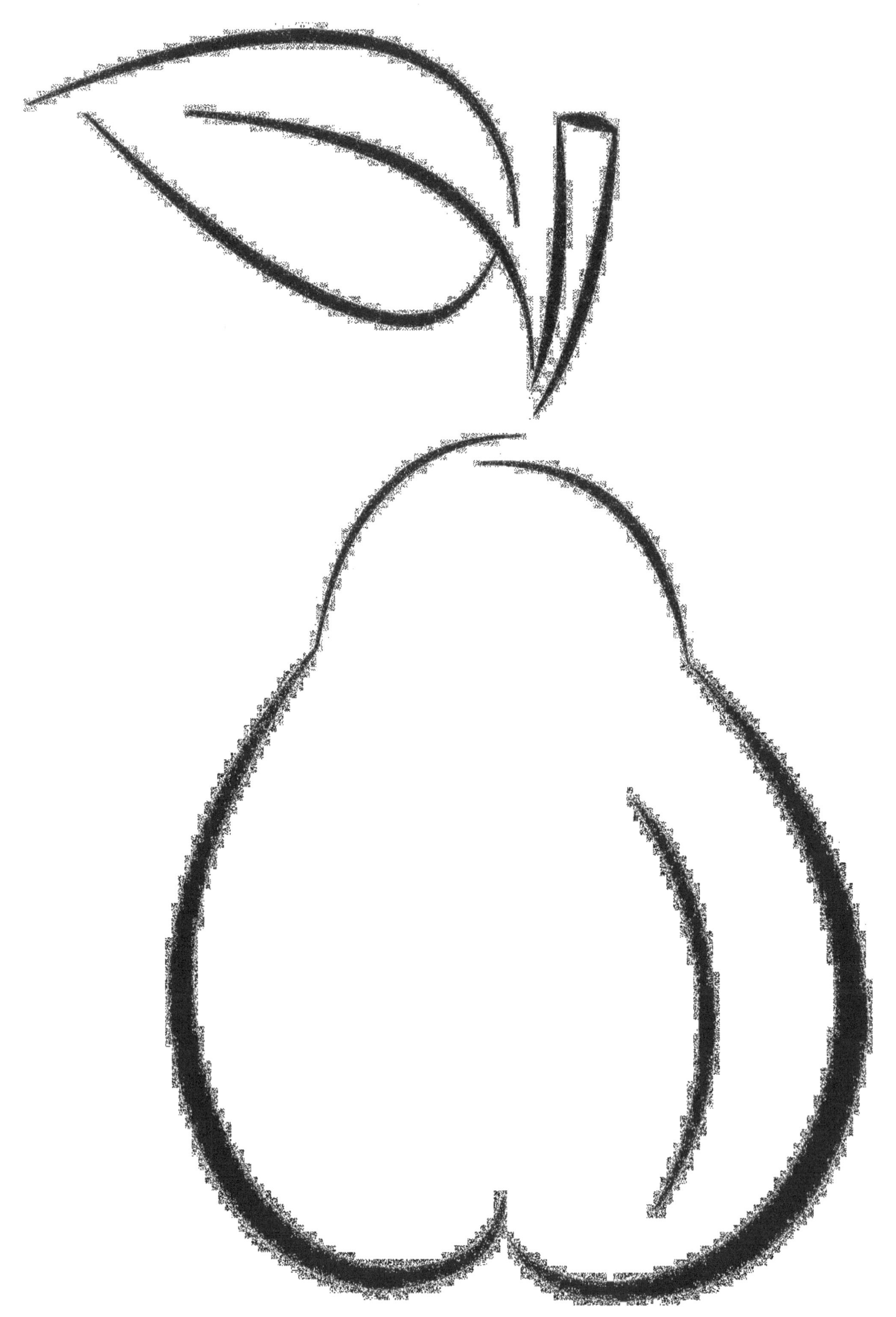

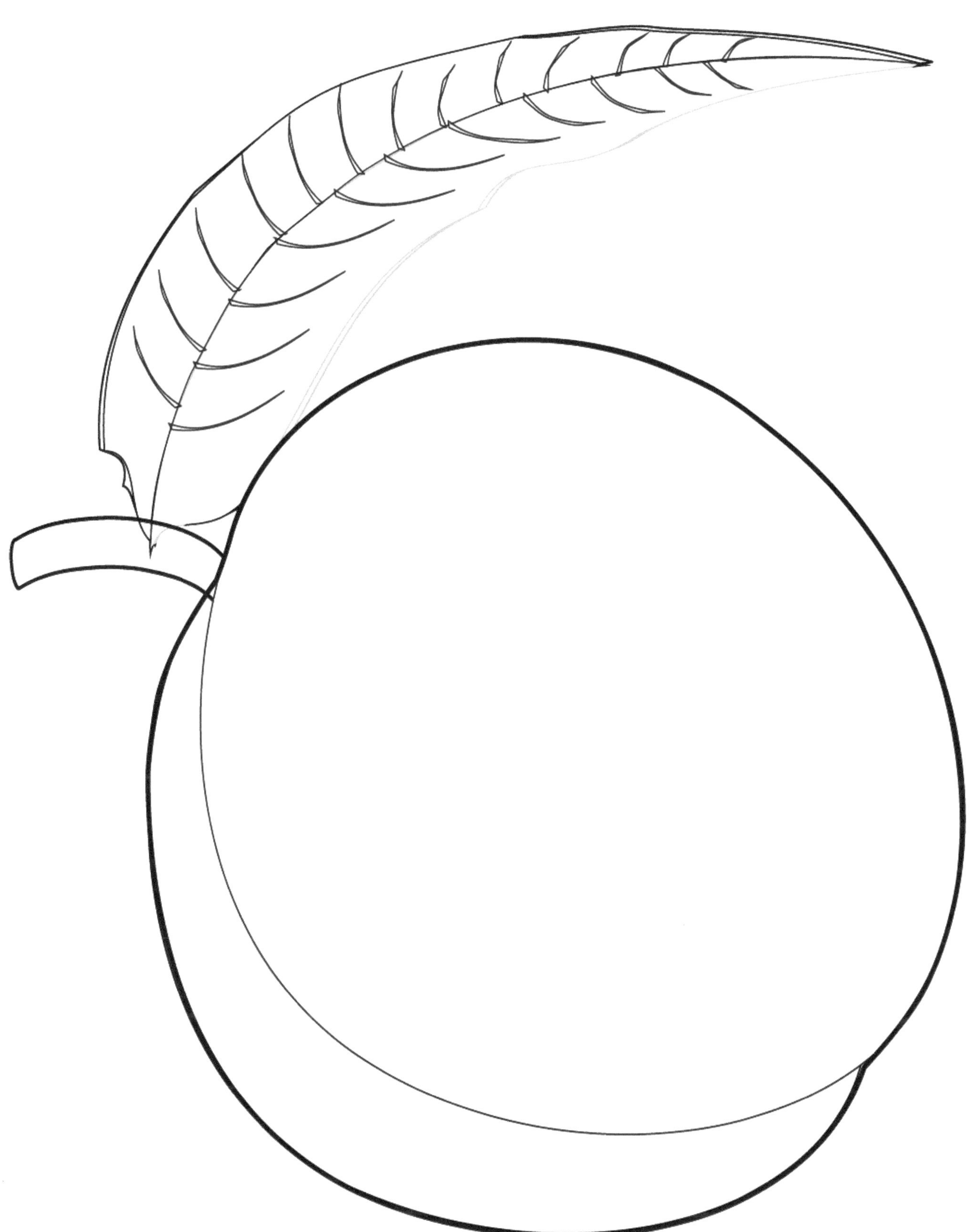

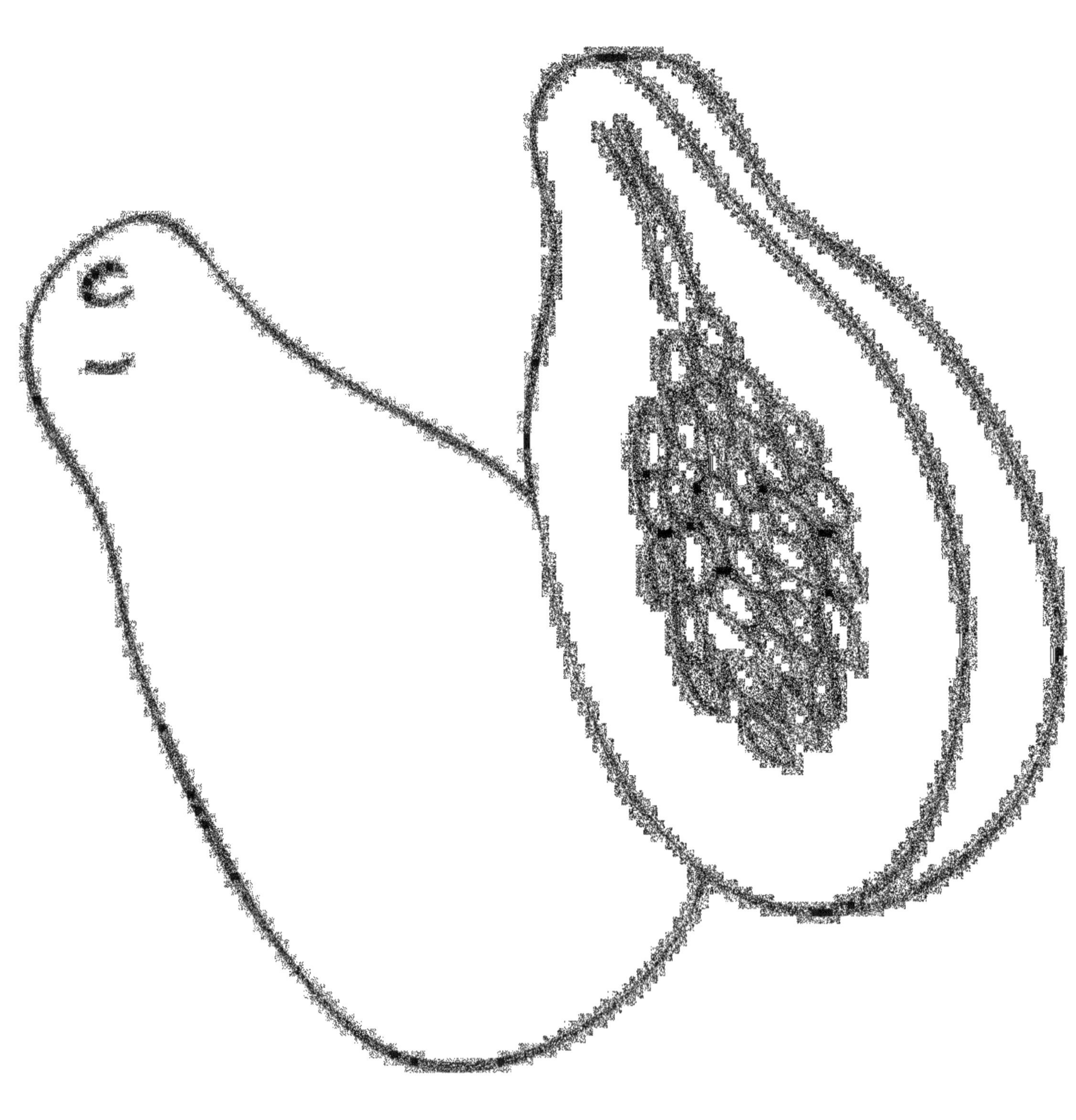

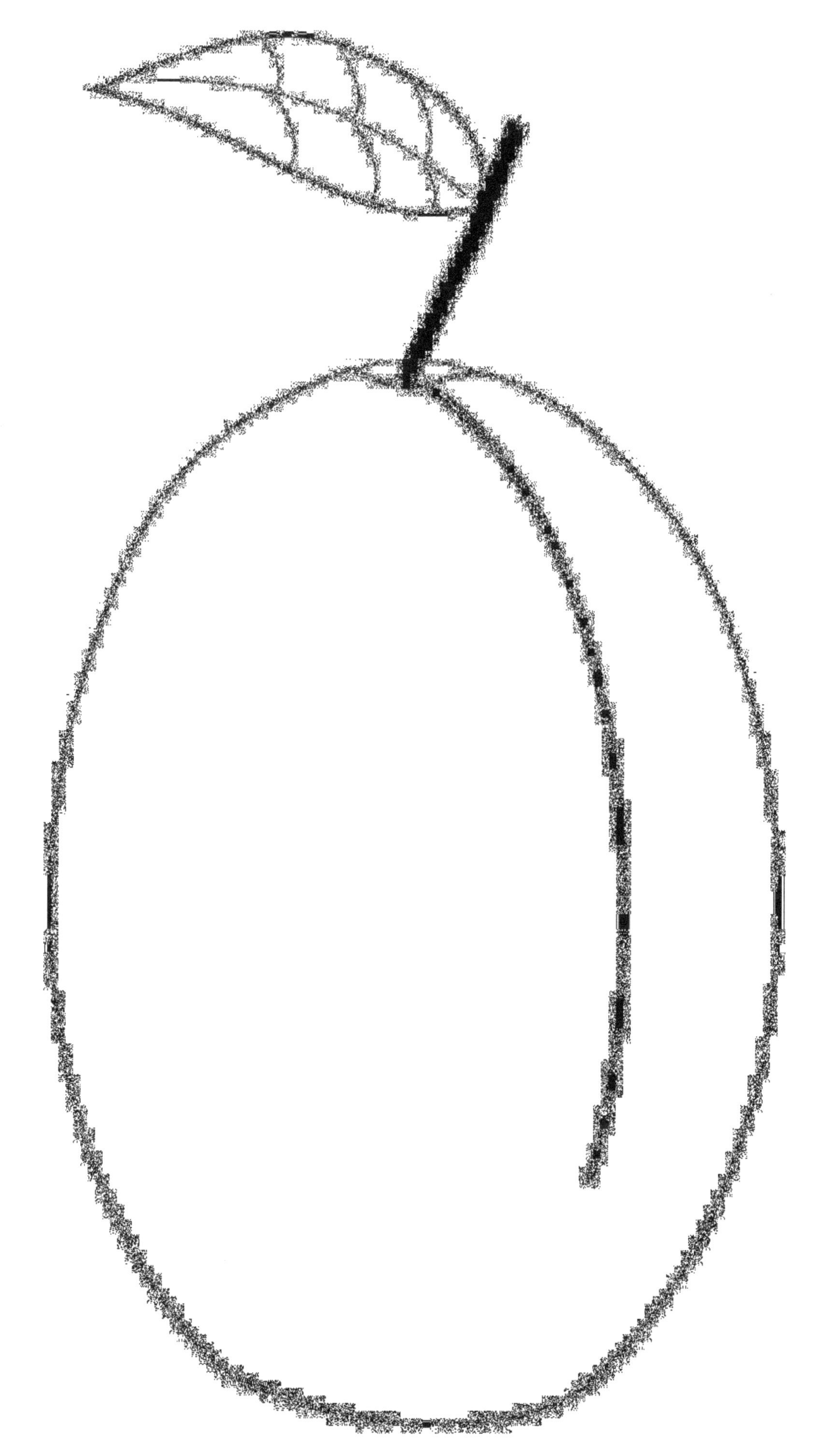

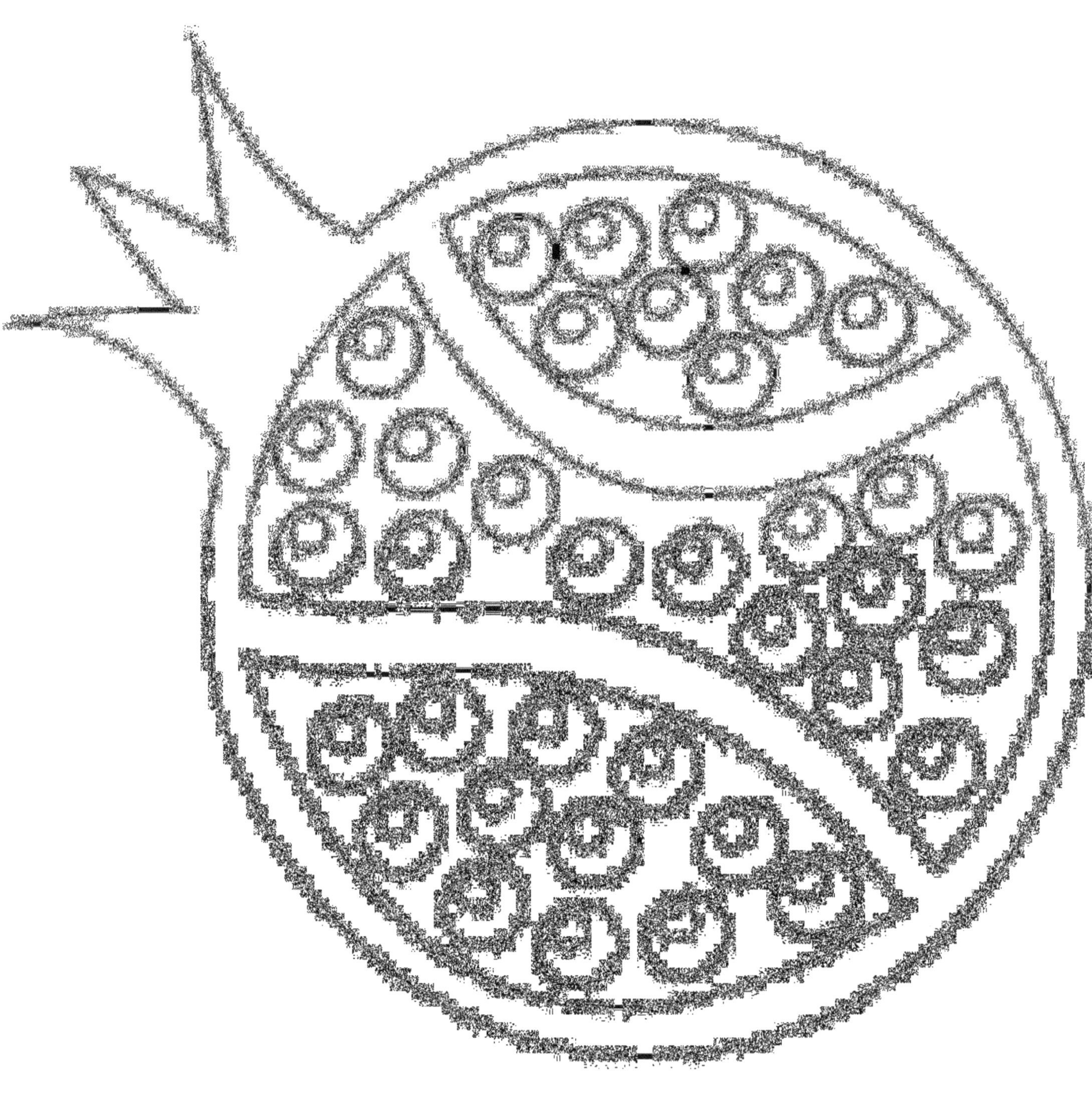

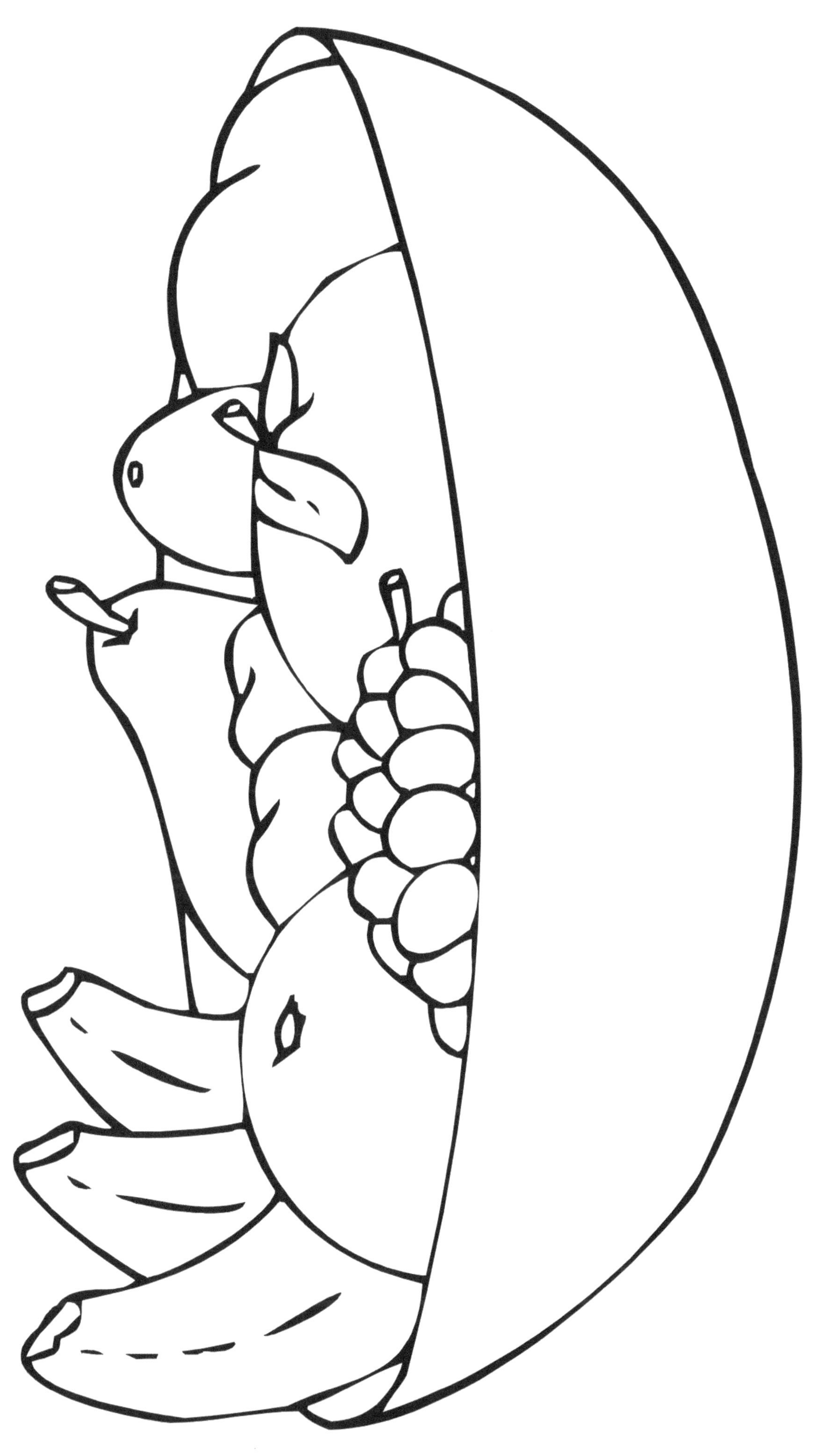

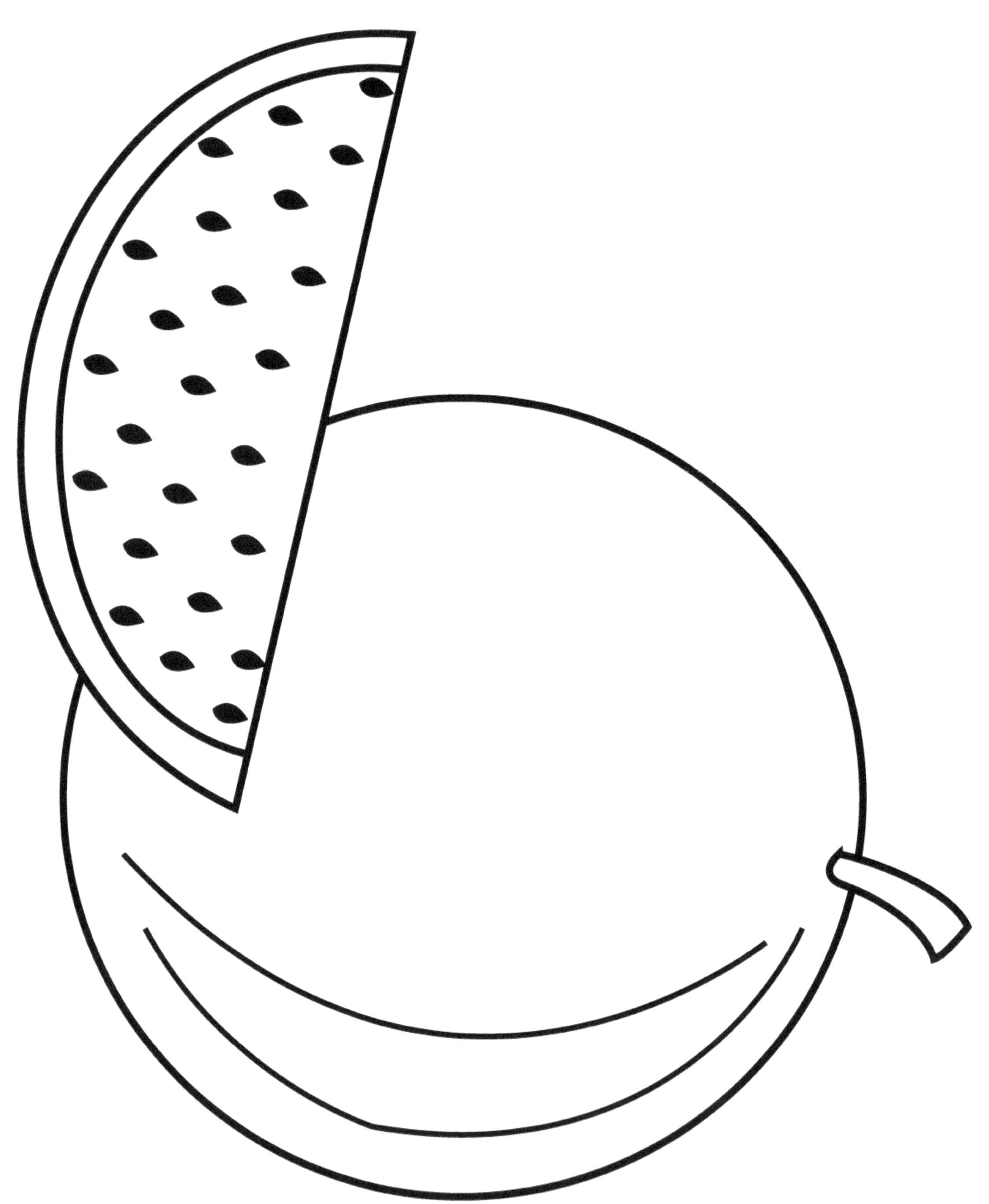

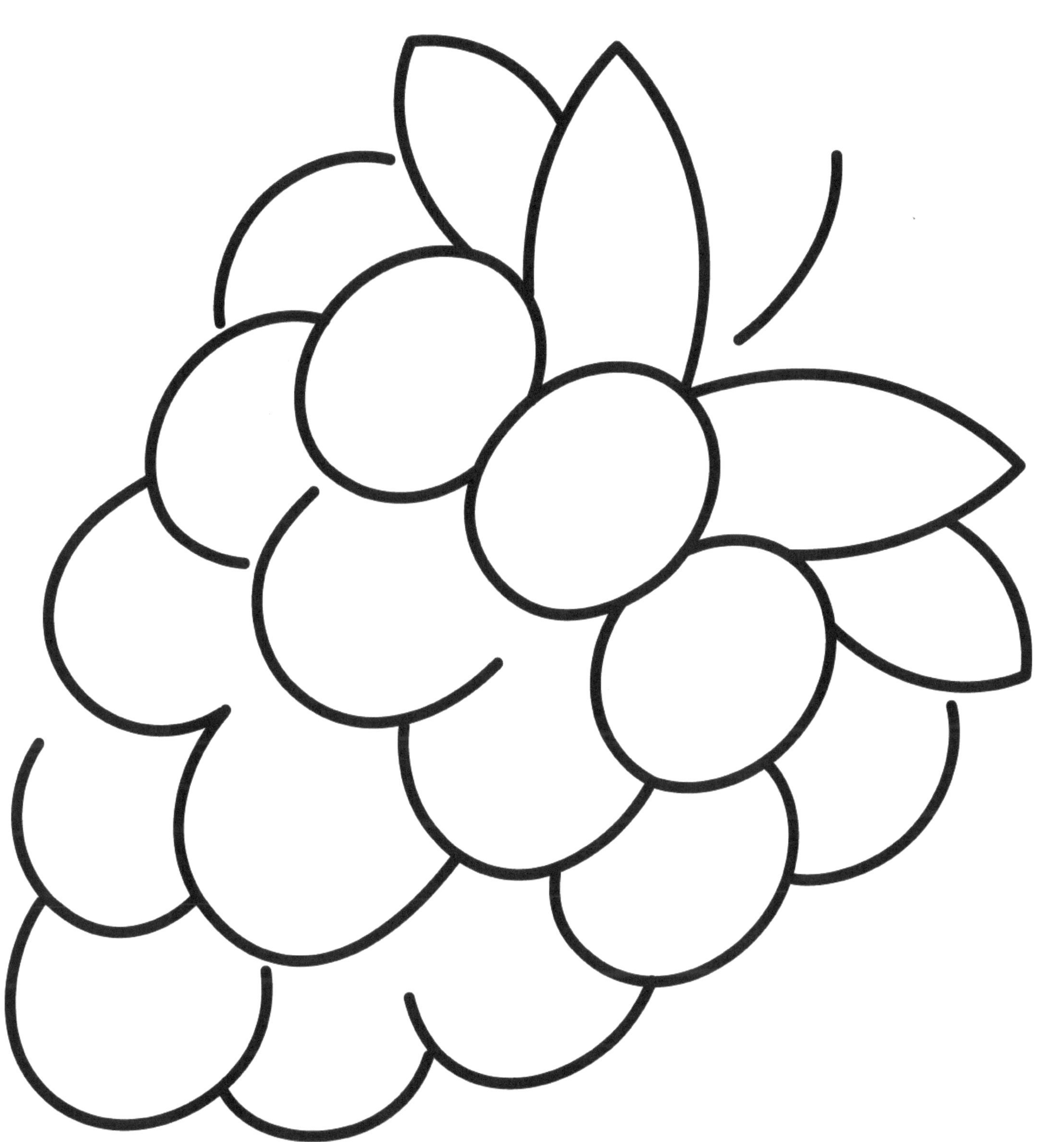

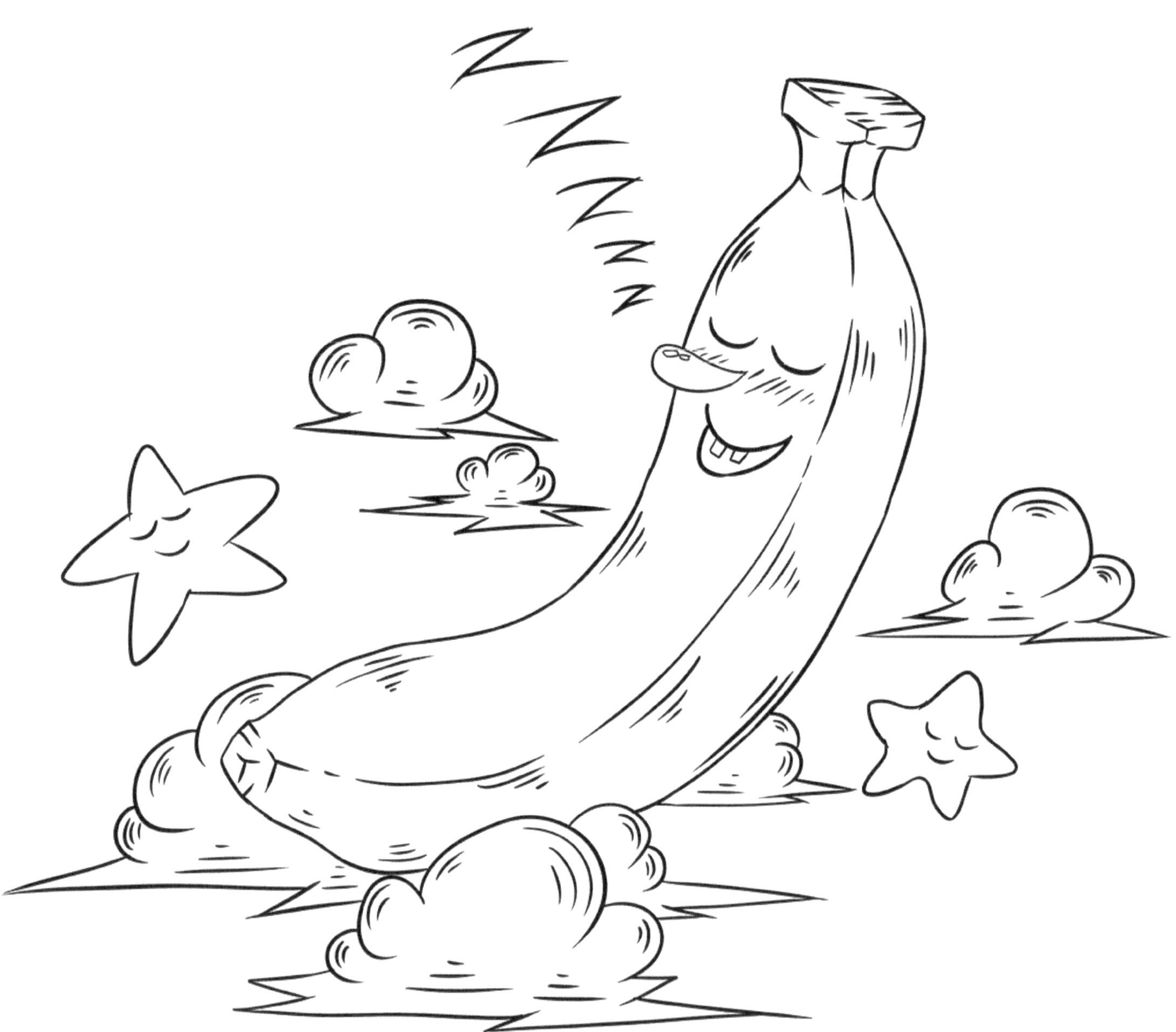

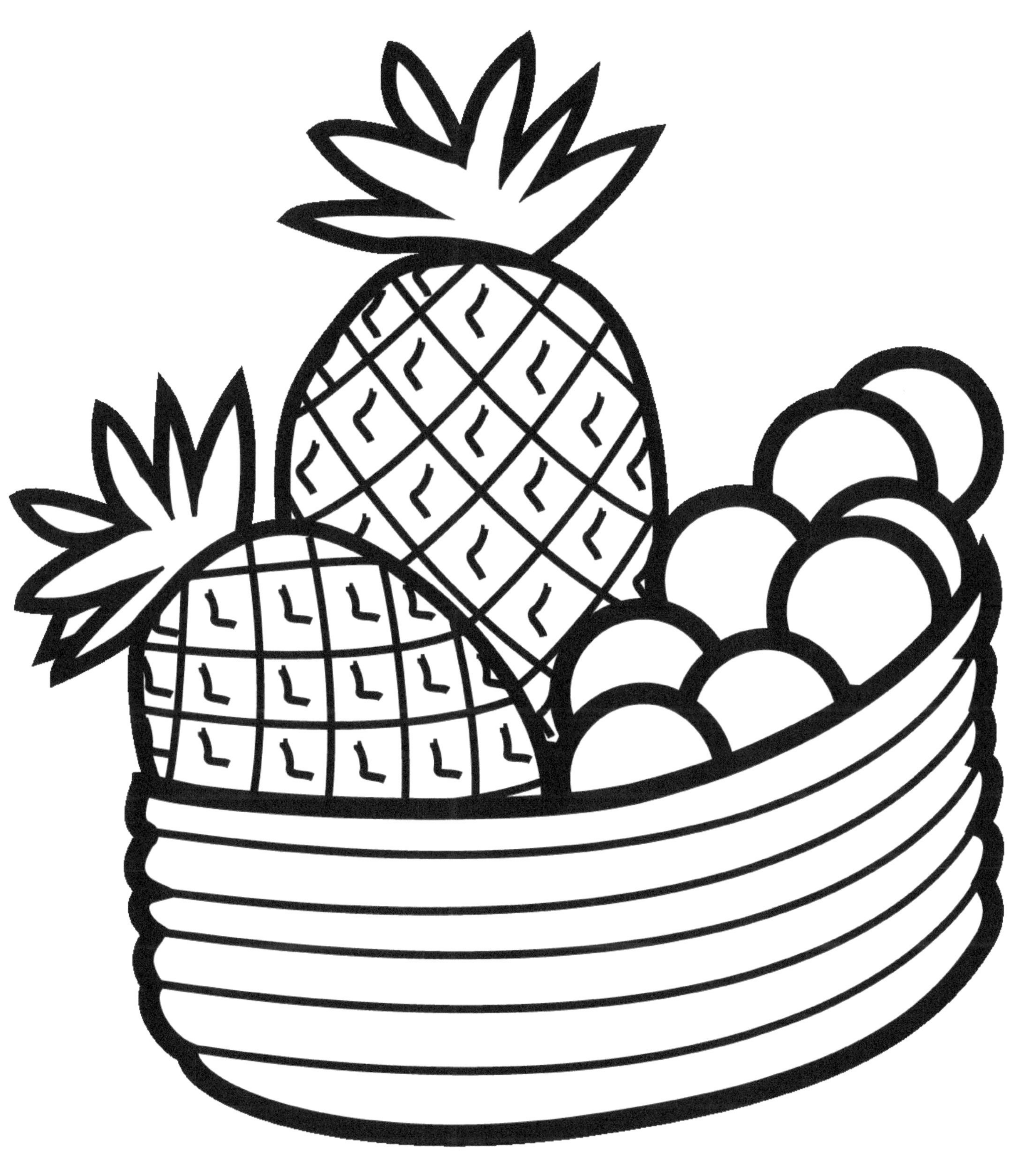